HOMEOPATHY FOR HEALTH

Comprehensive Guide To Natural Remedies, Holistic Healing, And Personalized Treatments For Optimal Wellness

DR. MELISSA STOTLER

Copyright © 2023 by Dr. Melissa Stotler

Disclaimer:

The data in this book, "Acupuncture Therapy Simplified," is solely meant to be informative and instructional.

This book is not intended to replace expert medical advice, diagnosis, or care. No medical, health, or other professional services are offered by the author, publisher, or any affiliated parties

Individual outcomes may differ in the practice of these therapies, which entail a variety of approaches and methodologies.

A one-on-one session with a trained or certified healthcare professional is still preferable. It is best to consult a trained healthcare provider before making any decisions regarding your health.

The author of this book is not affiliated with any specific website, product, or organization related to any of these therapies.

All reasonable measures have been taken by the author and publisher to guarantee the authenticity and dependability of the material contained in this book.

Contents

Homeopathy For Health is an essential guide for those seeking to integrate holistic healing practices into their wellness journey. This comprehensive book delves into the core principles of homeopathy, shedding light on its historical evolution, the foundational laws, and the philosophy that underpins this alternative medicine system. Readers will gain insight into the process of potentization and how homeopathic remedies are crafted and selected, emphasizing the art and science behind these remedies.

The book explores the application of homeopathy in treating both acute and chronic conditions. It provides an overview of how to address immediate health issues with commonly used remedies, detailing dosage and administration for effective relief. For chronic conditions, it offers strategies for long-term management, including remedy selection, treatment plans, and monitoring progress, supported by real-life case studies.

Emotional and mental health is another crucial focus, where the book explains the role of homeopathy in addressing anxiety, depression, and stress. Through case examples, it demonstrates the effectiveness of remedies for emotional well-being and explores how these remedies can complement other therapeutic approaches.

Special attention is given to the safe use of homeopathy for children and infants, with guidance on appropriate remedies, dosage adjustments, and addressing parental concerns. Additionally, the book covers women's health issues, including menstrual, menopausal, and postpartum care, along with remedies for hormonal imbalances.

The guide also highlights the role of homeopathy in promoting overall lifestyle and wellness, offering practical advice on integrating remedies into daily routines to enhance health and prevent issues. Readers will learn how to choose and work with a homeopath, prepare for consultations, and effectively communicate symptoms.

With detailed FAQs addressing common concerns, this book provides valuable answers on remedy selection, combining homeopathy with conventional treatments, and managing expectations for results. It stands as a comprehensive resource for anyone interested in harnessing the power of homeopathy for a healthier, balanced life.

CHAPTER ONE

PRINCIPLES OF HOMEOPATHY

Homeopathy is based on a set of principles that distinguish it from conventional medicine. At its core, homeopathy operates on the idea that "like cures like." This principle, known as the Law of Similars, suggests that a substance causing symptoms in a healthy person can be used to treat similar symptoms in a sick person. For instance, if a substance like onion causes watery eyes in a healthy individual, it could potentially be used to treat someone suffering from watery eyes due to a cold.

Another key principle is the Law of Minimum Dose, which posits that the lower the dose of a remedy, the more effective it becomes. Homeopathy utilizes highly diluted substances, often so diluted that no molecules of the original substance remain. This concept is based on the belief that these diluted remedies can stimulate the body's vital force to heal itself.

The holistic approach of homeopathy considers the individual as a whole rather than focusing solely on the symptoms of a disease. Homeopaths aim to understand the physical, emotional, and psychological state of a person, tailoring the remedy to address the overall condition rather than just isolated symptoms.

Historical Background

Homeopathy was developed in the late 18th century by Samuel Hahnemann, a German physician. Dissatisfied with the medical practices of his time, Hahnemann began experimenting with alternative treatments. His observations led him to the principle that a substance causing symptoms in a healthy person could be used to treat similar symptoms in illness. This foundational idea became known as the "Law of Similars."

Hahnemann's journey into homeopathy began with his translation of William Cullen's Materia Medica, where he noted that quinine, used to treat malaria, caused symptoms similar to malaria itself. This realization prompted him to experiment with the idea and eventually develop a systematic approach to treatment using highly diluted substances. His work, "Organon of Medicine," published in 1810, laid the groundwork for homeopathic theory and practice.

The practice of homeopathy spread across Europe and eventually to other parts of the world. Despite facing criticism and skepticism from mainstream medicine, homeopathy gained a significant following due to its unique approach and the successes reported by its practitioners and patients.

Founders And Key Figures

Samuel Hahnemann is recognized as the founder of homeopathy. His pioneering work and development of the fundamental principles of homeopathy shaped the practice as it is known today. Hahnemann's dedication to developing a more humane and effective system of medicine led him to create a comprehensive methodology that emphasized patient individuality and minimal dosages.

In addition to Hahnemann, several key figures have contributed to the development and popularization of homeopathy. One notable figure is James Tyler Kent, an American homeopath who expanded upon Hahnemann's work and is renowned for his contributions to the understanding and classification of homeopathic remedies. Kent's writings and teachings remain influential in homeopathic education.

Another important figure is Constantine Hering, known for his contributions to the field of homeopathy and his role in the establishment of homeopathic institutions in the United States. Hering's work included the development of the "Hering's Law," which describes the sequence of healing in homeopathic practice and emphasizes the importance of the body's natural healing process.

Fundamental Laws

Law of Similars

The Law of Similars is the cornerstone of homeopathy. It asserts that a substance causing symptoms in a healthy person can be used to treat those same symptoms in a sick person. This principle is based on the idea that remedies should mirror the symptoms of the illness to stimulate the body's healing mechanisms. For example, a remedy that induces a rash in a healthy individual might be used to treat a patient with a similar rash, aiming to prompt a healing response.

Law of Minimum Dose

The Law of Minimum Dose suggests that the more diluted a remedy, the more potent it becomes. Homeopathic remedies are prepared through a process of serial dilution and succussion (vigorous shaking), which is believed to enhance their therapeutic effects. This principle is rooted in the belief that even extremely diluted substances can have a profound impact on the body's vital force, thereby facilitating healing.

Understanding Potentization

Potentization is a process used in homeopathy to prepare remedies through serial dilution and succussion. The process begins by diluting a substance in water or alcohol. This diluted solution is then subjected to succussion, which involves vigorous shaking. This process is repeated multiple times, each time creating a more diluted solution.

The idea behind potentization is that it transfers the "energetic imprint" of the substance into the solution. Homeopaths believe that this imprint, rather than the chemical substance itself, has therapeutic value. Potentization is thought to activate the vital force or healing energy of the remedy, making it effective even at extremely low concentrations. This method contrasts sharply with conventional medicine, which often relies on the chemical properties of substances.

Homeopathic Philosophy

Homeopathic philosophy is rooted in the belief that health is a dynamic state of balance within the body, mind, and spirit. According to this philosophy, illness arises when this balance is disrupted. Homeopathy aims to restore this balance by stimulating the body's healing abilities rather than merely addressing symptoms.

Central to homeopathic philosophy is the concept of the "vital force," a vital energy that governs the body's health and healing processes. Homeopaths view disease as a disturbance in this vital force and believe that homeopathic remedies can help realign and restore balance to the vital force.

Homeopathic practice emphasizes treating the whole person, considering emotional and psychological states along with physical symptoms. This holistic approach seeks to understand the individual's unique symptoms and circumstances, leading to a more personalized and comprehensive treatment plan. This philosophy aligns with the belief that true healing involves more than just alleviating symptoms; it requires addressing the underlying causes and supporting overall well-being.

CHAPTER TWO

HOMEOPATHIC REMEDIES

Homeopathic remedies are based on the principle of "like cures like." This means that a substance that causes symptoms in a healthy person can when diluted and prepared in a specific way, treat similar symptoms in a sick person. These remedies are derived from natural sources, including plants, minerals, and animal substances. They are prepared through a process called potentization, which involves repeated dilution and succussion (vigorous shaking).

Homeopathic remedies aim to stimulate the body's natural healing processes. These remedies are used to address a wide range of health issues, from chronic conditions to acute illnesses. Each remedy is tailored to match the specific symptoms and overall state of the individual, rather than treating a disease in isolation.

Types Of Remedies

Homeopathic remedies come in various types, each suited to different conditions and treatment approaches. The most common types include:

Single Remedies: These are made from a single substance, such as a plant or mineral. Single remedies are used to address specific symptoms or conditions. For example, Arnica montana is often used for bruising and trauma.

Combination Remedies: These remedies contain a blend of several single remedies formulated to treat a range of symptoms or conditions. They are often used for common ailments or to support general health.

Complex Remedies: Similar to combination remedies, complex remedies consist of multiple substances, but they are formulated based on a specific condition or symptom profile. They are designed to address more complex health issues or multifaceted symptoms.

Remedy Preparation Process

The preparation of homeopathic remedies follows a meticulous process to ensure their effectiveness. The steps include:

Source Collection: The initial material, such as a plant, mineral, or animal substance, is collected. This material is used to create the mother tincture.

Mother Tincture Preparation: The collected material is combined with alcohol or another solvent to extract its medicinal properties. This mixture is then allowed to steep for a specific period.

Potentization: The mother tincture undergoes a series of dilutions and succussions. Each dilution involves mixing a small amount of the tincture with a larger volume of alcohol or water. The mixture is then vigorously shaken. This process is repeated multiple times to achieve the desired potency.

Final Preparation: The potentized remedy is then prepared in its final form, such as pellets, tablets, or liquid. These forms are used for administration to the patient.

Commonly Used Remedies

Several homeopathic remedies are widely used due to their effectiveness in treating various conditions. Some commonly used remedies include:

Arnica montana: Known for its use in treating bruising, muscle soreness, and trauma. It is often recommended after physical injuries or surgery.

Belladonna: Used for conditions with sudden onset of symptoms, such as high fever, headaches, and inflammation. It is also helpful for conditions with throbbing or pulsating pain.

Nux vomica: A remedy for digestive issues, including nausea, indigestion, and constipation, often linked to stress or overindulgence.

Rhus tox: Effective for joint and muscle pain, especially when it worsens with initial movement and improves with continued motion.

How Remedies Are Selected

Selecting the appropriate homeopathic remedy involves a thorough assessment of the patient's symptoms, overall health, and individual characteristics. The process includes:

Symptom Analysis: The homeopath evaluates the specific symptoms experienced by the patient, including their nature, duration, and triggers.

Patient History: An in-depth review of the patient's medical history, lifestyle, and emotional state is conducted to understand the full context of their health issues.

Constitutional Assessment: The homeopath considers the patient's overall constitution, including their physical, emotional, and mental characteristics, to choose a remedy that matches their total health picture.

Remedy Matching: Based on the collected information, the homeopath selects a remedy that best corresponds to the patient's symptoms and overall state.

Remedy Repertory And Materia Medica

In homeopathy, the Repertory and Materia Medica are essential tools for remedy selection and understanding.

Repertory: This is a comprehensive reference book that lists symptoms and the remedies associated with them.

It helps homeopaths identify potential remedies based on the patient's symptom profile.

The Repertory is organized systematically, making it easier to find the remedies that match specific symptoms.

Materia Medica: This is a detailed compilation of information about each homeopathic remedy, including its preparation, uses, and effects on the body.

It provides insights into the characteristics of remedies and helps in understanding how they can be applied to various conditions. The Materia Medica is used alongside the Repertory to confirm the suitability of a remedy for a given symptom pattern.

CHAPTER THREE

HOMEOPATHY FOR ACUTE CONDITIONS

Overview Of Acute Conditions

Acute conditions are sudden and severe medical issues that require prompt attention. These conditions typically manifest quickly and can include anything from a cold or flu to more intense symptoms like an asthma attack or a sudden injury.

Homeopathy offers a complementary approach to managing these conditions, focusing on the body's natural ability to heal itself.

In homeopathy, the aim is to treat the person as a whole rather than just addressing the symptoms.

This means considering the individual's overall health, emotional state, and specific symptoms to determine the most appropriate remedy.

Homeopathy operates on the principle of "like cures," where substances that cause symptoms in a healthy person are used in diluted form to treat similar symptoms in a sick person.

Common Acute Remedies

Homeopathy provides a variety of remedies for common acute conditions. Here are a few widely used remedies:

Aconite (Aconitum napellus): Often used for sudden onset of conditions, particularly those triggered by shock or trauma. It's helpful for symptoms that appear suddenly, such as anxiety or a high fever.

Belladonna (Atropa belladonna): Useful for conditions with intense, throbbing pain and high fever. It is often recommended for sudden, inflammatory conditions like tonsillitis or ear infections.

Arnica (Arnica montana): Known for its effectiveness in treating injuries, bruises, and strains. It's particularly helpful for reducing pain and bruising after a fall or trauma.

Nux Vomica (Strychnos nux-vomica): Used for conditions resulting from overindulgence in food or alcohol.

It can help with symptoms such as nausea, indigestion, and irritability.

Apis Mellifica (Apis mellifica): Best for conditions involving swelling and stinging pain, such as insect bites or allergic reactions. It can reduce inflammation and alleviate discomfort.

Dosage And Administration For Acute Conditions

In homeopathy, the dosage and administration of remedies depend on the specific condition and individual symptoms. Here's a general guide:

Potency: Remedies come in various potencies (e.g., 6C, 30C). For acute conditions, lower potencies like 6C or 30C are often used. Higher potencies might be reserved for more chronic or deep-seated issues.

Frequency: For acute conditions, remedies are usually taken more frequently at the onset of symptoms. For example, you might take a remedy every 15-30 minutes until symptoms improve. Once improvement is noted, the frequency can be reduced.

Form: Homeopathic remedies are commonly available in pillules, liquid drops, or tablets. Follow the instructions provided with the remedy or consult a homeopathic practitioner for guidance.

Administration: Place the remedy under the tongue and allow it to dissolve. Avoid eating or drinking for at least 15 minutes before and after taking the remedy to ensure optimal absorption.

Case Studies Of Acute Conditions

Case Study 1: Acute Cold

A 35-year-old woman developed a cold with a sudden onset of sneezing, a runny nose, and a scratchy throat. She took Aconite for the initial shock of her symptoms and Allium Cepa for the runny nose and sneezing. Her symptoms improved significantly within a few days, demonstrating the effectiveness of early intervention with homeopathic remedies.

Case Study 2: Sprained Ankle

A teenage athlete sprained her ankle during a game, experiencing immediate pain and swelling. She used Arnica to reduce the swelling and Rhus Toxicodendron to alleviate the pain and stiffness. With regular application, her recovery was swift, and she was back to her activities sooner than expected.

Case Study 3: Food Poisoning

A middle-aged man suffered from nausea, vomiting, and stomach cramps after a meal. Nux Vomica was administered to address the symptoms caused by overindulgence. The remedy helped alleviate his discomfort and stabilize his digestion, demonstrating the remedy's efficacy in acute digestive issues.

When To Seek Professional Help

While homeopathy can be effective for managing acute conditions, there are instances when professional medical help is necessary. Seek medical attention if:

Severe Symptoms: Symptoms are severe, persistent, or worsening despite homeopathic treatment. For example, if a high fever does not subside or if there is significant difficulty breathing.

Underlying Health Issues: Some pre-existing medical conditions or complications may be exacerbated by the acute condition.

Uncertain Diagnosis: The symptoms are unusual or the diagnosis is unclear. It's important to get a professional assessment to ensure proper treatment.

Chronic or Recurring Issues: If the acute condition recurs frequently or evolves into a chronic issue, a medical professional's intervention may be required for a comprehensive treatment plan.

In such cases, homeopathy can be used alongside conventional medicine to support overall health and recovery. Always consult with a healthcare provider to ensure the best approach to managing acute conditions.

CHAPTER FOUR

HOMEOPATHY FOR CHRONIC CONDITIONS

Identifying Chronic Conditions

Homeopathy can be a valuable approach to managing chronic conditions, which are typically long-lasting and persistent. Identifying these conditions involves recognizing symptoms that persist over time and significantly impact daily life. Common chronic conditions include arthritis, asthma, diabetes, and chronic fatigue syndrome.

The first step in identifying a chronic condition is to look for symptoms that are consistent and do not resolve with standard treatments. For example, chronic arthritis may cause ongoing joint pain and stiffness, while asthma might present as frequent breathing difficulties. It's essential to document these symptoms accurately, noting their frequency, intensity, and any factors that seem to trigger or alleviate them.

Homeopathic practitioners often perform a comprehensive assessment that includes reviewing medical history, current symptoms, and overall health status. This holistic view helps in selecting the most appropriate homeopathic remedies.

Common Chronic Remedies

Homeopathy offers a range of remedies tailored to different chronic conditions. Some commonly used remedies include:

Rhus Toxicodendron: Often used for arthritis with symptoms like stiffness and pain that worsen with rest and improve with movement.

Sulfur: Helpful for chronic skin conditions such as eczema, especially when the skin is dry and itchy.

Arsenicum Album: Used for chronic respiratory issues like asthma, particularly when there is anxiety and restlessness associated with the condition.

Calcarea Carbonica: Often recommended for chronic fatigue and conditions where there is weakness, anxiety, and excessive perspiration.

Each remedy is selected based on the individual's specific symptoms and overall health profile.

It's crucial to consult with a qualified homeopath to determine the most suitable remedy for your condition.

Treatment Plans For Chronic Conditions

Developing a treatment plan for chronic conditions in homeopathy involves a tailored approach. The plan typically includes:

Initial Consultation: A detailed assessment of the patient's health, including their medical history and current symptoms. This helps the homeopath understand the condition in its entirety.

Remedy Selection: Based on the consultation, a specific homeopathic remedy is chosen. The selection process considers both the physical symptoms and the emotional or psychological state of the patient.

Dosage and Administration: Homeopathic remedies are administered in specific potencies and dosages. The homeopath will prescribe the appropriate dosage and frequency based on the condition and the patient's response.

Follow-Up Appointments: Regular follow-up appointments are essential to monitor the patient's progress and adjust the treatment plan as needed. This ensures that the remedy continues to be effective and that any changes in symptoms are addressed promptly.

Lifestyle and Dietary Recommendations: Homeopathic treatment often includes suggestions for lifestyle and dietary changes that can support the overall healing process.

Monitoring Progress

Monitoring progress is a critical aspect of homeopathic treatment for chronic conditions. It involves:

Symptom Tracking: Keeping a detailed record of symptoms, including any changes in frequency, intensity, or duration. This helps in assessing how well the remedy is working.

Regular Reviews: Scheduled follow-up visits with the homeopath to review progress. These visits allow for adjustments to the treatment plan based on the patient's feedback and symptom changes.

Evaluating Effectiveness: Assessing whether the symptoms are improving, worsening, or staying the same. This evaluation helps in determining if the current remedy is still appropriate or if a different approach is needed.

Adjusting Treatment: Based on progress reviews, the homeopath may adjust the remedy or dosage to better address the evolving symptoms.

Long-Term Management Strategies

Long-term management of chronic conditions with homeopathy involves a proactive and ongoing approach:

Consistent Treatment: Adhering to the prescribed treatment plan and attending regular follow-up appointments. Consistency is key to managing chronic conditions effectively.

Lifestyle Adjustments: Implementing lifestyle changes recommended by the homeopath, such as dietary modifications, stress management techniques, and exercise routines.

Preventive Measures: Engaging in preventive measures to reduce the risk of symptom flare-ups.

This may include avoiding known triggers or implementing supportive practices that enhance overall well-being.

Ongoing Evaluation: Continuously evaluating the effectiveness of the treatment plan and making necessary adjustments. Long-term management requires periodic reassessment to ensure that the approach remains suitable.

Patient Education: Educating patients about their condition and the role of homeopathy in managing it. This empowers patients to actively participate in their treatment and make informed decisions about their health.

By following these strategies, individuals with chronic conditions can achieve better management and improved quality of life through homeopathic treatment.

CHAPTER FIVE

HOMEOPATHY FOR EMOTIONAL AND MENTAL HEALTH

Homeopathy offers a unique approach to treating emotional and mental health issues, focusing on balancing the mind and body through individualized remedies. This holistic system of medicine is based on the principle of "like cures like," meaning that substances causing symptoms in a healthy person can when prepared homeopathically, cure similar symptoms in a sick person.

Role Of Homeopathy In Mental Health

Homeopathy plays a significant role in mental health by addressing the underlying emotional and psychological causes of mental health issues rather than merely alleviating symptoms. Homeopathic remedies aim to restore balance to the mind and body, supporting overall mental wellness. By treating the person as a whole, rather than focusing solely on the mental illness, homeopathy seeks to promote emotional resilience and well-being.

Personalized Treatment

Homeopathic treatment is highly individualized. Practitioners consider a person's overall health, lifestyle, and emotional state to prescribe a remedy that matches their specific needs. This personalized approach helps address the root causes of mental health issues and supports long-term emotional stability.

Holistic Approach

Homeopathy treats the whole person rather than just the symptoms. This holistic approach is designed to restore balance in the emotional and mental realms, enhancing a person's overall sense of well-being.

Remedies for Anxiety, Depression, and Stress

Homeopathy offers a range of remedies specifically formulated to address anxiety, depression, and stress. Each remedy is selected based on an individual's unique symptoms and emotional state.

Anxiety

For anxiety, remedies such as Argentum Nitricum, Aconite, and Gelsemium can be helpful. Argentum Nitricum is often used for anxiety with anticipatory fears, while Aconite may be chosen for sudden and intense anxiety following a traumatic event.

Gelsemium is suited for anxiety accompanied by trembling and weakness.

Depression

In cases of depression, remedies like Natrum Muriaticum, Sepia, and Staphysagria may be effective.

Natrum Muriaticum is commonly prescribed for individuals who feel a deep sense of sadness and isolation, while Sepia can help those who feel overwhelmed and emotionally detached. Staphysagria is used for depression related to suppressed emotions and indignation.

Stress

To manage stress, remedies such as Nux Vomica, Phosphorus, and Silica are often recommended. Nux Vomica is suitable for stress caused by overwork and irritability, while Phosphorus is used for stress with a tendency to be overly sensitive. Silica can be helpful for stress accompanied by physical exhaustion.

Case Examples And Effectiveness

Understanding the effectiveness of homeopathy in emotional and mental health can be enhanced through real-life case examples.

Case Example 1: Anxiety Relief

A patient experiencing severe anxiety with symptoms of restlessness and palpitations found relief through Aconite. After a traumatic event, this remedy helped alleviate the intense fear and agitation, allowing the patient to regain a sense of calm.

Case Example 2: Depression Management

Another patient suffering from long-term depression and feelings of deep sadness benefited from Natrum Muriaticum. The remedy helped to lift the overwhelming sadness and improve emotional stability, enabling the patient to engage more fully in daily activities.

Case Example 3: Stress Reduction

For a person dealing with high levels of stress due to a demanding job, Nux Vomica was prescribed. This remedy helped reduce irritability and improve the individual's ability to manage stress more effectively, resulting in improved overall well-being.

Understanding Emotional Symptoms

Accurate identification of emotional symptoms is crucial for effective homeopathic treatment. Emotional symptoms can manifest in various ways, including mood swings, irritability, sadness, and anxiety. By understanding these symptoms in detail, homeopathic practitioners can tailor remedies to address the specific emotional state of the individual.

Identifying Symptoms

Recognizing the nuances of emotional symptoms involves noting their intensity, duration, and impact on daily life. For instance, is the sadness persistent or situational? Does the anxiety occur in specific situations or all the time? Detailed symptom assessment helps in selecting the most appropriate remedy.

Emotional Patterns

Understanding emotional patterns, such as recurring themes or triggers, provides insight into the underlying causes of emotional distress. This information is essential for choosing remedies that align with the individual's emotional profile and overall health.

Combining Homeopathy with Other Therapies

Homeopathy can be effectively combined with other therapies to enhance overall treatment outcomes. Integrating homeopathy with conventional medicine, psychotherapy, or lifestyle changes provides a comprehensive approach to managing emotional and mental health.

Complementary Approaches

Homeopathy can complement conventional treatments by addressing aspects of mental health that may not be fully covered by traditional methods. For example, homeopathic remedies can support emotional healing alongside psychotherapy, offering a holistic approach to mental wellness.

Integrative Strategies

Integrative strategies involve combining homeopathic remedies with lifestyle changes, such as stress management techniques, exercise, and healthy eating. This holistic approach supports emotional and mental health by addressing multiple aspects of well-being simultaneously.

Professional Guidance

It is important to consult with both a qualified homeopathic practitioner and other healthcare professionals when combining therapies. This ensures a coordinated approach to treatment and helps to maximize the benefits of each therapy while avoiding potential interactions or conflicts.

CHAPTER SIX

HOMEOPATHY FOR CHILDREN AND INFANTS

Homeopathy is often considered for treating various health issues in children and infants due to its gentle and holistic approach. Understanding how to use homeopathy effectively in this age group involves recognizing the differences in their physiological needs and responses compared to adults.

Safe Use Of Homeopathy In Children

When using homeopathy for children and infants, safety is paramount. It's essential to choose remedies that are specifically formulated for young patients. Homeopathic remedies are highly diluted, which generally makes them safe, but it's crucial to follow guidelines for use. Always consult with a pediatric homeopath or healthcare provider before starting any treatment to ensure it's appropriate for your child's specific condition.

Common Remedies For Pediatric Issues

Several homeopathic remedies are commonly used to address pediatric issues. For example:

Chamomilla: Often used for teething pain or irritability. It can help soothe a child who is restless, irritable, and in pain.

Belladonna: Useful for high fevers with sudden onset, especially when accompanied by redness and heat.

Apis Mellifica: Helps with swelling and redness, often used for insect bites or allergic reactions.

Pulsatilla: Suitable for children who are weepy, clingy, and have symptoms that shift or change frequently.

These remedies are chosen based on specific symptoms and individual characteristics, so it's important to consult a professional for personalized recommendations.

Dosage Adjustments For Different Ages

Dosage in homeopathy is often adjusted based on the child's age and weight. Infants and young children typically require lower doses compared to older children and adults.

Infants (0-2 years): Generally, a lower potency (e.g., 6C or 30C) is used, and doses are given less frequently. Remedies may be administered in the form of a liquid or dissolved in water.

Children (2-12 years): Potencies of 6C to 30C are commonly used, and doses may be increased slightly depending on the severity of symptoms. Tablets or granules can be used, but it's important to adjust the dosage to the child's weight and response.

Adolescents (12 years and older): Potencies similar to those used for adults (e.g., 30C or 200C) may be appropriate, but dosage should still be adjusted based on the individual's needs and the specific issue being addressed.

Addressing Parental Concerns

Parents often have concerns about the efficacy and safety of homeopathic treatments. Common questions include:

Is it safe? Homeopathic remedies are typically very safe due to their high dilution, but consulting a healthcare provider ensures that the remedy is suitable for your child's specific condition.

How do I know it's working? Improvement in symptoms, even gradual, can indicate that the remedy is having an effect. It's important to monitor the child's response and adjust treatment as needed.

What if symptoms worsen? If symptoms worsen or do not improve, it's important to seek medical advice. Homeopathic remedies should not replace conventional medical treatment for serious conditions.

Case Studies In Pediatric Homeopathy

Case studies can provide valuable insights into how homeopathy is used to address various conditions in children. For instance:

Teething Pain: A case study might describe a child who experienced significant relief from teething pain using Chamomilla, illustrating the remedy's effectiveness in calming irritability and reducing discomfort.

Frequent Colds: Another study may detail a child who suffered from frequent colds and benefited from a specific homeopathic protocol, leading to a decrease in the frequency and severity of infections.

Behavioral Issues: A case might explore how a remedy like Pulsatilla helped a child with emotional issues, such as anxiety or clinginess, highlighting how homeopathy can address behavioral and emotional aspects.

These case studies demonstrate the practical application of homeopathy and its potential benefits for various pediatric issues, offering real-life examples of how remedies can support children's health and well-being.

CHAPTER SEVEN

HOMEOPATHY FOR WOMEN'S HEALTH

Homeopathy offers a holistic approach to women's health, focusing on treating the whole person rather than just isolated symptoms. This system of medicine uses natural substances in highly diluted forms to stimulate the body's healing processes. For women, homeopathy can be a gentle and effective option to address various health concerns throughout different stages of life.

Common Women's Health Issues Addressed

Women experience a range of health issues unique to their physiology. Homeopathy provides remedies for common conditions such as:

Menstrual Irregularities: Irregular cycles, heavy bleeding, or painful menstruation can be managed with remedies like Pulsatilla or Sepia, tailored to individual symptoms and emotional states.

Menopausal Symptoms: Hot flashes, mood swings, and insomnia associated with menopause can benefit from remedies like Lachesis or Sulphur, which address both physical and emotional symptoms.

Reproductive Health Problems: Conditions like ovarian cysts or fibroids may be supported with remedies such as Kali Carbonicum or Thuja, considering both the physical manifestations and the overall health of the patient.

Understanding these issues in detail helps in choosing the right remedy, as homeopathy treats based on the complete symptom profile and individual constitution.

Remedies For Menstrual And Menopausal Symptoms

Menstrual Symptoms: For menstrual cramps, remedies like Magnesia Phosphorica can provide relief from spasmodic pain. If the menstrual flow is excessively heavy, Ferrum Phosphoricum might be recommended to help restore balance and reduce blood loss.

Menopausal Symptoms: Homeopathic remedies for menopause vary based on individual experiences. For persistent hot flashes, remedies such as Lachesis or Sanguinaria might be suggested. Sepia is often used for mood swings and irritability, while Cimicifuga can help with joint pain and muscular issues related to menopause.

Each remedy is chosen based on the overall symptom picture, including emotional and physical aspects, and is tailored to the specific needs of the individual.

Pregnancy And Postpartum Care

During pregnancy and postpartum periods, homeopathy can offer support for a variety of issues:

Pregnancy: Remedies like Nux Vomica and Sepia can address common pregnancy symptoms such as nausea, fatigue, and digestive issues. For concerns like back pain or swelling, remedies like Rhus Toxicodendron or Apis Mellifica may be helpful.

Postpartum Care: After childbirth, remedies like Arnica Montana can assist in recovery from physical trauma and bruising. For emotional challenges like postpartum depression, remedies such as Staphysagria or Ignatia may be used, depending on the emotional state and specific symptoms.

Homeopathic remedies are selected based on the specific needs of the new mother and her recovery process, aiming to support both physical and emotional well-being.

Hormonal Imbalances And Remedies

Hormonal imbalances can lead to a variety of symptoms, including irregular periods, mood swings, and weight changes. Homeopathy addresses these imbalances through remedies that align with the individual's specific symptoms and overall health:

Premenstrual Syndrome (PMS): Remedies like Agnus Castus or Calcarea Carbonica can be used to manage symptoms like irritability, bloating, and mood swings.

Thyroid Issues: For hypothyroidism or hyperthyroidism, remedies such as Iodum or Lycopus may be recommended based on the symptoms and underlying causes.

Adrenal Fatigue: Remedies like Gelsemium or Phosphoric Acid can help support adrenal function and alleviate symptoms of fatigue and stress.

Choosing the right remedy involves a comprehensive understanding of the symptoms and the patient's overall health.

Case Examples In Women's Health

Case 1: Menstrual Cramps: A woman experiencing severe menstrual cramps with nausea and mood swings was treated with Pulsatilla. Her symptoms improved significantly, with reduced pain and more stable moods during her menstrual cycle.

Case 2: Menopausal Hot Flashes: A patient suffering from frequent hot flashes and night sweats found relief with Lachesis. Her symptoms became less intense, and her sleep quality improved.

Case 3: Postpartum Recovery: After a traumatic childbirth, a new mother received Arnica Montana for bruising and Arnica's mental strain. Her recovery was smoother, with reduced soreness and a better emotional state.

These examples illustrate how homeopathy can be tailored to individual needs, providing relief and support for various women's health issues.

CHAPTER EIGHT

HOMEOPATHY FOR LIFESTYLE AND WELLNESS

Homeopathy is not just about treating ailments; it's also a powerful tool for enhancing lifestyle and overall wellness. By addressing the root causes of health issues and promoting balance, homeopathic remedies can support a more vibrant and fulfilling life.

Using Homeopathy For Daily Wellness

Incorporating homeopathy into daily wellness routines can help maintain balance and prevent illness. Homeopathic remedies, tailored to individual needs, offer a natural approach to supporting overall health. Remedies like Arnica montana can help with minor injuries and muscle soreness, while Natrum muriaticum can assist in managing stress and emotional imbalances. Regular use of these remedies can support a balanced lifestyle and contribute to long-term wellness.

Remedies For Lifestyle-Related Issues (Diet, Sleep)

Homeopathy offers targeted remedies for common lifestyle-related issues such as diet and sleep disturbances. For digestive issues linked to diet, remedies like Nux vomica can alleviate symptoms of indigestion and bloating, while Carbo vegetabilis can help with gas and discomfort. When it comes to sleep, remedies such as Coffea cruda can address sleeplessness due to an overactive mind, and Pulsatilla can aid those who experience restless sleep due to emotional factors. By choosing remedies based on specific symptoms, you can support your body's natural healing processes and maintain better health.

Enhancing Overall Health With Homeopathy

To enhance overall health, homeopathy focuses on improving the body's innate ability to heal itself.

Remedies like Sulphur can be beneficial for individuals dealing with chronic skin conditions, while Thuja can help with immune system support and detoxification.

Regular consultations with a homeopathic practitioner can help tailor remedies to your unique needs, ensuring that you are addressing both physical and emotional aspects of your health.

Incorporating lifestyle changes such as balanced nutrition and regular exercise, alongside homeopathic remedies, can further boost your overall well-being.

Preventive Measures And Remedies

Preventive care is a cornerstone of homeopathy, aiming to maintain health and prevent illness before it arises. Remedies such as Oscillococcinum are often used to prevent flu-like symptoms, while Echinacea can support immune function during cold and flu season. Additionally, regular use of remedies like Calendula can promote skin health and aid in healing minor cuts and abrasions. By integrating these preventive measures into your routine, you can reduce the risk of illness and support a healthier lifestyle.

Integrating Homeopathy Into Daily Life

Integrating homeopathy into daily life involves more than just taking remedies; it's about making holistic changes that support your well-being. Start by incorporating remedies that align with your specific health goals, such as stress management or digestive health.

Create a routine that includes time for relaxation and self-care, and consider keeping a journal to track your progress and any changes in your health. By making homeopathy a regular part of your life, you can enhance your overall health and well-being in a natural and balanced way.

CHAPTER NINE

COMMON CONCERNS AND DETAILED FAQS

How Do I Choose The Right Remedy For My Condition?

Choosing the right homeopathic remedy can feel overwhelming, but understanding the basic principles of homeopathy can simplify the process. Homeopathy operates on the principle of "like cures like," meaning that a remedy that causes symptoms in a healthy person is used to treat similar symptoms in a sick person.

Start by identifying your primary symptoms and any emotional or physical changes you've experienced. Homeopathic remedies are selected based on a comprehensive picture of your symptoms, including any unique characteristics. For example, if you have a cold with a lot of sneezing and a runny nose, a remedy like Allium Cepa might be recommended. If your symptoms are more along the lines of a cough with a tickle in the throat, Phosphorus might be a better fit.

Consulting a qualified homeopath can be beneficial as they can provide a detailed analysis and suggest remedies tailored specifically to your needs. If you prefer to self-treat, consider using well-regarded homeopathic materia medica or guides that describe remedies for common ailments and their specific indications.

Can Homeopathy Be Used Alongside Conventional Treatments?

Yes, homeopathy can be used alongside conventional treatments. Many people find that combining homeopathy with conventional medicine can provide complementary benefits.

Homeopathic remedies are generally safe and non-toxic, which makes them a gentle option to support overall well-being and alleviate symptoms.

However, it is important to inform all of your healthcare providers about any homeopathic remedies you are using to avoid potential interactions with conventional medications. Homeopathy focuses on treating the whole person rather than just the symptoms, which can complement conventional treatments by addressing underlying imbalances and enhancing the body's healing process.

If you are under the care of a physician for a serious condition, discuss the use of homeopathy with them to ensure it fits well with your treatment plan. Combining approaches can often help manage symptoms more effectively and improve overall health outcomes.

What Should I Do If My Symptoms Get Worse?

If your symptoms worsen after starting homeopathic treatment, it's important to take a measured approach. First, assess any recent changes or additional factors that might be influencing your condition. Sometimes, initial worsening can occur as part of a healing process called "proving," where symptoms briefly intensify before improvement.

Contact your homeopath or healthcare provider to discuss the changes. They may suggest adjusting the remedy or dosage or selecting a different remedy that better matches your updated symptoms. In cases where symptoms escalate significantly, seeking conventional medical advice is also recommended to rule out any serious underlying issues or complications.

Keep track of your symptoms and any other changes in your health, and communicate this information to your healthcare providers to ensure that you receive the most appropriate care and adjustments to your treatment plan.

How Do I Know If A Remedy Is Genuine?

Ensuring that you use a genuine homeopathic remedy involves a few key practices. First, purchase remedies from reputable suppliers or pharmacies that specialize in homeopathic products. These sources often adhere to strict standards for quality and authenticity.

Check for proper labeling on the remedy, including the remedy name, potency, and expiration date. Authentic homeopathic remedies are typically labeled with a name that corresponds to a substance used in homeopathy and are prepared according to established homeopathic practices.

If you're unsure about the authenticity of a remedy, consult with a professional homeopath or pharmacist who can verify the product's quality. Avoid purchasing remedies from unverified online sources or stores without a clear reputation in the homeopathic community.

How Long Will It Take To See Results?

The time it takes to see results from homeopathic treatment can vary widely depending on several factors, including the nature of the condition, the individual's overall health, and the remedy chosen. Some people may notice improvements within a few days, while others might take several weeks.

Homeopathy aims to stimulate the body's natural healing processes, so gradual improvement is often expected. In acute conditions, such as a cold or minor injury, relief can be relatively quick. For chronic conditions, it may take more time to see significant changes, as the treatment works to address deeper imbalances.

Patience and consistency are key. Follow the guidance of your homeopath and allow time for the remedy to work. Regular follow-up appointments can help monitor progress and make necessary adjustments to the treatment plan, ensuring that you are on the right path to recovery.